Health and Faith

Shelisskia V. Melton

Health and Faith
Copyright © 2013by **Shelisskia V. Melton**

Dedication

This book is dedicated to YOU!!!!
Now is the time to start living a healthy lifestyle while building your faith. Reading this book is no accident!!! God knew that you would be reading the guidelines from this book at this very moment to help improve your lifestyle.

This book is dedicated to Keith Bivens who has inspired me to go forth with my dream about writing this book. Keith also designed the beautiful book cover along with the pictures in the book.   I would like to thank him for his support and guidance.

This book is also dedicated to my boss, Dr. Carl Brutkiewicz and his wife Barbara Brutkiewicz. I won't ever forget when I first told Dr. Brutkiewicz that I was going to write this book. I asked him did he think that I could write a book while he was going into a patient's room. He stopped, turned around and looked at me and immediately said yes. Thanks for always believing in me! I also thank you for being a great role model and a Dr. who passionately cares about his patients.

This book is also dedicated to my Pastor, Elder Stephen C. Shaw and his wife Laniece Shaw. Thanks for always teaching about our faith walk with God. I can remember you telling me, "The way has already been made." Day by day I walk in faith and not by sight. Thanks for instilling the word faith in me. By faith this book has been written. To God Be the Glory!!!

This book is dedicated to my entire family, especially my two lovely daughters, Paige B. Melton and Porschia B Melton and my loving parents Samuel Melton, Jr. and Bertha J. Melton.

things not seen.   For by it the elders obtained a good
testimony. By faith we understand that the worlds were
framed by the word of God, so that the things which are
seen were not made of things which are visible.

Praying, trusting in God, believing in God, and know
that you will receive it in Jesus name is faith. Know
that God works in the natural, as well as, in the Super-
natural. As you have a closer walk with God through
prayer, praise, and worship by being obedient to His
word, living righteous, and having that personal
relationship with God you will know that he is Lord.
Have faith in knowing that the only thing that will
cleanse you is God's word.

Because of who you are **Lord** I give you the Honor.
Because of who you are **Lord** I give you the Praise.
Because of who you are **Lord** I Worship you. Because
of who you are **Lord** I Lift up my voice and sing.
Jehovah- Jireh you are my provider **Lord** you reign!

References

Roger-Pamplona, George D., M.D. Encyclopedia of Foods and Their Healing Power (1995).

Perricone, Nicholas, M.D. 7 Secrets to Beauty, Health, and Longevity (2006)

Yeager, Selene. The Doctors Book of food Remedies (2007)

Holy Bible, King James Version, Hand Size Giant Print Reference Bible

Broadman & Holman, Holman Concise Bible Dictionary (1997)

American Academy of Family Physicians, Information from your family doctor (2010)

Foreword

Shelisskia Melton has been a nursing assistant in my office for over two years. I have been in family practice in the same location for over 20 years and I must say that Shelisskia has been the most optimistic and upbeat employee I have ever had or could even imagine. I have reviewed her guidelines on health and living and totally agree with all that she has written.

Shelisskia's positive attitude is an asset to my practice. The patients receive from her, hope, encouragement, a caring listener when they are having troubles and leave having made a friend who passionately wants them to get better and lead healthier lives.

Shelisskia leads by example. Every time I see what she is eating I can tell it is quite healthy and she treats her body as a temple. Her strong religious faith is infectious to all, including her co-workers as well as her boss.

Shelisskia entered the medical field at mid career, however I think she has found her calling and I am certain that over the many years of her medical career she will have a positive impact on many, many lives.

Carl Brutkiewicz, M.D.

Foreword

In a world of ever changing thoughts on living healthy both spiritual and naturally we find the church silent on the natural man and at ease on faith. I applaud Shelisskia in her endeavor to enlighten the people of God with this book.

I have known Shelisskia for over 7 years and have had the pleasure of being her Pastor for 6 plus years. I find her to be a person of unfailing faith for such a work as this. We are in a time of ever failing health and also failing faith in God in America.

I pray this book will open new doors for all that reads it as it has done for me. May the anointing of Jesus Christ be upon the author of this awesome work!

Pastor Stephen C. Shaw

Preface

I became interested in writing this book many years ago. I decided to change my life for the better. By changing my life for the better I knew that I had to put God first in everything I did. It was a daily process and determination to change for the better. I had to cry out to God and repent. After crying to God and repenting I had no desire to live the way I lived. God immediately removed the thing that I desired to do that was wrong in my life.

I made the decision on my own to live a healthy life style by eating healthy and exercising. First, I had to change my people, places and things. I started to be around positive people. People who lived a life with morals, and values, as well as integrity,(Christians). I had to choose positive places to go, and positive things to do. I hung around People who I could learn and grow from. I surrounded myself with people who knew more than me.

By living a positive and a healthy life I knew I had to always pray and worship God. The God of Abraham, Isaac, and Jacob (Let's be clear)!!! I also had to read God's word daily. Seeking him and mediating on his word day and night. While being obedient. I went to Wednesday night bible study, Sunday school (It was a working process), and Church. Also, getting active in church.

I knew I had to come back to my roots. Meaning when I was a little child my mom and dad kept us in church. I can recall going to Church on Sunday mornings, 3oclock Church services, BTU, and lest not leave out night services. And please lest night forget about 2 weeks of Vacation Bible School during the summer. I had big fun being with my friends and looking forward to drinking as much cool-aid as I wanted and eating cookies. My mom, Bertha J. Melton, was the Vacation Bible School Director for over 25 years at Union Missionary Baptist Church in Plateau, Al. on Bay Bridge Rd.

I had a great childhood. I was surrounded by love, discipline, laughter and loving family members and friends. I went to a private school from the 1st thru 8th grade at St. James Major, in Prichard, Al. From the 9th thru 12th grade I went to C.F. Vigor High where I graduated. I attended the University of Mobile and received a B.A. degree in Sociology and a minor in Psychology. In my later years I went into the Medical Field. I have 2 lovely daughters Paige Beretta Melton and Porschia Bianca Melton.

There are 2 roads in life to choose from. The positive road, or the negative road which is the road to destruction. This book will show you the positive ways to live a healthy lifestyle and it will also show you what will happen if you choose the road to destruction by living an unhealthy lifestyle. I hope you will enjoy this book and it will change your life for the better. **Good Better Best never let them rest until your Good is Better and your Better is Best!!!!!!!**

Table of Contents

Introduction **11**

Health and Faith **13**

Chapter1: Rejuvenating the body and mind **15**

    Getting plenty of sleep rejuvenates our body and mind 15

    Health benefits of sleep 16

    Benefits of drinking water 16

    Benefits of eating fruits and vegetables 18

    Benefits of nuts... 18

    Good Protein 19

    Benefits of grains 19

    Benefits of olive oil 20

Chapter 2: How to look younger and feel great with the proper nutrients and vitamin power **22**

    Nutrients for the body 22

    Vitamins for the body 22

    Antioxidants.. 25

Chapter 3: Choosing your foods wisely will promote better health for your body and can help you live a healthy lifestyle **28**

    Diabetes 28

    Hypertension (high blood pressure) 30

Cholesterol 31

What are the good and bad types of cholesterol? 31

Alzheimer's Disease 32

Headaches 34

Strokes... 34

Heart Attacks (disease) 36

Chapter 4: Faith.. **38**

References **42**

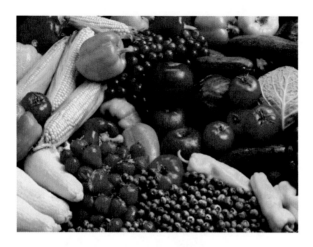

Introduction

Our health depends on the many small decisions that we make each day to have a better lifestyle. The decisions we make affects our health and have to do with the foods we eat. We must decide which foods to eat and how they are best prepared. It is vital to understand the foods well in order to select those that maintain our health, and those that treat various diseases. After reading this book you will live a better lifestyle, and have better understanding that all foods are not equal.

All foods provide nutrients and energy. There are harmful foods, and beneficial foods, some can cause disorders and diseases; while others can bring healing and health to our bodies. I am glad to show you in this book how the foods that we eat can help fight diseases. Certain foods we eat have the healing power to reverse heart disease, bad cholesterol level, diabetes, strokes, Alzheimer's disease, headaches, and hypertension (high blood pressure).

Also, know that we have to have faith in order for us to succeed in life. Remember that our bodies are a living sacrifice holy and acceptable unto God. We must watch what we put in our bodies. How can we look, and feel great if we put harmful and toxic foods and drinks in our bodies? There is no way that we can look, and feel great!!! Faith without works is dead. And dead faith is worse than no faith at all. Faith must work; it must produce; it must be visible. Verbal faith is not enough; mental faith is insufficient. Faith must be there, but it must be more. Remember that faith must inspire action. You must develop endurance to live a healthy lifestyle, and a lifestyle that's filled with faith.

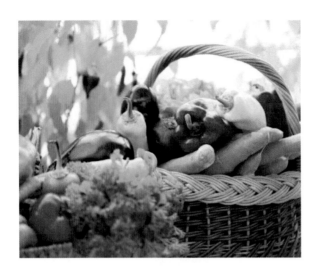

HEALTH AND FAITH

Our bodies are a living sacrifice holy and acceptable unto God. We must be in tuned with our bodies. It's time to watch our diets in how we are eating and drinking. Getting the proper nourishment in our bodies are essential for our health. How we look and feel plays a major role in our life. If we feel great we look great!

The 7 keys to rejuvenating the body are: **Getting plenty of sleep**, drinking at least 8 glasses of **water** a day, **eating fruits and vegetables**, **nuts**, good **protein, grains**, and unsaturated fats such as **olive oil**. If we don't take these 7 keys to rejuvenate our body into consideration there will be a major breakdown in our health and strength. Rejuvenating the body will help the organs, cells, brain, etc. function properly. Did you know by getting the proper **nutrients**, **vitamins** and

antioxidants in your body will make you look younger and feel wonderful? Did you also know that choosing your foods wisely plays a great part in **diabetes, hypertension (high- blood pressure), cholesterol, Alzheimer's Disease, headaches, strokes, heart attacks etc.?**

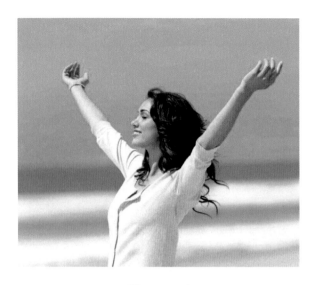

Chapter 1

Rejuvenating the body and mind

Getting plenty of sleep rejuvenates our body and mind.

It is so important that our bodies get enough sleep and rest. Our bodies have to recover from the daily stress we put on it. When you are deprived from sleep this runs your immune system down and you will end up sick. With the proper rest and sleep your daily duties are performed with a clear head. Also, your daily functions and the way we age are determined by how much rest and sleep we get. Sleep deprivation can lead to becoming irritable. Getting enough sleep affects our physical and mental health.

Did you know that drowsiness is the brain's last step before falling asleep? If you are driving while being drowsy it can lead to an accident. Studies make it clear that sleep deprivation is dangerous. Individuals who are sleep deprived who perform hand coordination and eye coordination test perform as badly or worse than those who are intoxicated.

Health benefits of sleep:

- **Improves memory** - Dr. Rapport says " if you are trying to learn something, whether it's physical or mental, you learn it with a certain point with practice". In other words if you are trying to learn something new, whether it's playing softball or learning how to sew you'll perform better after sleeping.
- **Live longer** - Sleep affects the quality of life. If you sleep better, you can live better. Illnesses may affect sleep patterns too.
- **Improves inflammation**- Inflammation is linked to diabetes, heart disease, stroke, premature aging and arthritis. People who get less than six hours of sleep at night have higher blood levels of inflammation.

Benefits of drinking water:

Lose weight: All you need is water! Water is a healthy way to feel full without going in for a second helping. Drinking more water can help you lose weight. Water washes away weight! Drinking water is a great way to cure hunger pangs. When we are thirsty, we think it's time to eat. When drinking water with meals you take in fewer calories. Drinking water about 20 minutes before meals reduces the amount of calories a person eats.

Fatigue: Not getting enough water can cause fatigue. Many individuals think of fatigue as being caused by not getting enough sleep or actually working too hard. Energy levels start to decline when cells throughout your body are not getting enough water. To quench their thirst, they draw water from the bloodstream. The blood is thick and harder to pump. The extra work causes the energy levels to decline.

Improve the Brain: Drinking water is one of the best ways to keep your brain sharp. Lack of water affects your focus and memory ability. Not getting enough water can cause the mind to get fuzzy. Our thirst mechanism slows down as we age, so we are not aware that we need water. When we don't get enough water we get dehydrated, and severe dehydration brings on mental confusion.

Improves Skin: Drinking water keeps your skin looking good. Dehydration makes your skin look more dry and wrinkled. Water replenishes skin. Your cells absorb water and increases moisture and elasticity.

Digestion: Without enough water you will suffer from irregularity and constipation. Water helps remove wastes from the body by keeping the stools soft to prevent constipation. A strong digestive system is critical for our body to absorb nutrients that it needs. Constipation may lead to colon cancer. Stools become hard and dry when you don't drink enough water, and it takes them longer to move through your system.

Benefits in Eating Fruits and Vegetables

Fruits and vegetables have many vitamins and minerals that help you stay healthy. Fruits and vegetables are good for your body and health. Eating a diet rich in fruits and vegetables helps lower blood pressure, reduces the risk of heart disease and some cancer. Try to aim for about 9 servings of fruits and vegetables a day. Choose your color variety of dark green, red, yellow, and orange.

Fruits and vegetables contain natural antioxidant that fights Free Radicals. People who eat a vegetarian diet gain protection from diseases, and live healthier, longer lives. Oranges contain four potent antioxidants. Other antioxidant foods are strawberries, citrus fruits, and nuts.

Benefits of Nuts

- Nuts provide energy and are very nutritious.
- They do not cause obesity.
- They are a healthy alternative to meat given their richness in protein, vitamins, and minerals.
- They can be eaten raw.
- They protect the heart by reducing the risk of a heart attack.
- They do not provide uric acid.

Good Protein

Protein makes you feel full after eating and keeps you full for hours. Good protein has the unique power to satisfy hunger. Meats are among the best sources of protein. If you don't want to eat meat, you can also get protein from fish, beans, nuts, and grains. All nuts are rich in protein, and they contain a generous supply of vitamins and minerals. Peanuts are the highest in protein of any nut. Peanuts contain all the essential amino acids we can't do without. The protein in peanuts is a complete protein. Walnuts, almonds, brazile nuts, cashews are a good source of protein. Beans are a healthy alternative to meat. Like red meat beans are loaded with protein. Beans are a great source of vitamins and minerals.

Benefits of Grains:

- **They are rich in fiber**: This insoluble fiber acts like a broom by sweeping the digestive tract.
- **They prevent diabetes.** Research shows that insoluble fiber plays a role in diabetes prevention. Insoluble fiber is found in whole grain products. The more whole grain products are eaten, the lower the risk of non-insulin dependent diabetes. Diabetics tolerate whole-grain products better than those of refined grains.
- **They reduce cancer risk** in the breast and colon, when whole grains are eaten on a regular basis.

- **They help avoid coronary disease and arteriosclerosis**. The protective effects of whole grains regarding cardiovascular disease are due to high levels of: unsaturated fatty acids (in the germ), and antioxidants.
- **They help avoid constipation.** Intestinal function improves by eating whole grains. They increases and accelerates fecal volume and passage through the intestines, and they facilitates the elimination of bile acids which are toxic substances.
- **They produce a sense of satiety** because of their fiber content. The fiber swells in the stomach. When the fiber swells in the stomach, this helps reduce additional food intake which can cause obesity.
- **They contain no cholesterol**, and contribute to the reduction level in the blood.

Benefits of Olive Oil:

- Promotes heart health. Olive oil protects against coronary disease (myocardial infarction and angina) with regular consumption.
- It serves as mild laxative. It helps avoid constipation when it is taken on an empty stomach (1 to 2 tablespoons).
- It controls cholesterol level. Olive oil does not reduce total cholesterol as much as seed oils. The use of olive oil provides greater protection and arteriosclerosis and coronary disease than any other oil.

Olive oil is a better fat from butter and margin. Yet it contains almost the same number in calories. They behave differently inside the body. Saturated fats are found mainly in meats and dairy foods. Saturated fat blocks arteries and raises the risk of heart disease. Olive oil is a monounsaturated fat. With no more than 2 grams of saturated fat per tablespoon, olive oil is recommended by the American Heart Association for your food preparation.

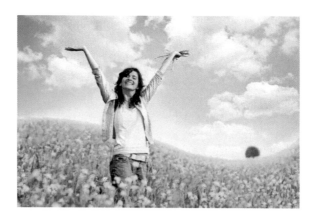

Chapter 2
How to look younger and feel great with the proper nutrients and vitamin power.

Nutrients for the Body:

According to the U.S. Department of Health and Human Services, the key to loosing fat and maintaining a healthy weight is the calorie. Calories are the fuel we burn to keep going. When we have too many calories we store them as fat. There are 3,500 calories to a pound. We have to make sure we put the proper nutrients and vitamins in our diet. If not our bodies will gradually slow down.

Vitamins for the Body

Vitamin A

- **Vitamin A is good for your teeth**. Vitamin A is used to form dentin, a layer of bone like material beneath the surface of the teeth. One of the best ways to get vitamin A is eating foods high in beta-carotene, such as carrots, Yellow-orange squash, and kale. Sweet potatoes are a great source of vitamin A.

- **Vitamin A is good for the eyes.** It helps block the effects of free radicals. Vitamin A is a powerful antioxidant. You can get lots of vitamin A by eating apricots. Vitamin A helps vision by forming a pigment that the eye needs in order to be able to see in dim light. People with low levels of vitamin A may suffer from night blindness. Night blindness makes it difficult to drive after dark. The beta-carotene in carrots helps improve and protect vision.
- **Vitamin A is good for the skin.** Vitamin A helps the lining of your digestive system, and the lining of your lungs. It's a barrier against germs that's trying to enter your body. Raw asparagus is a good source of vitamin A.

Vitamin B6 and B12

- **Vitamin B6 and B12 are good for memory problems.** The B vitamins help keep your mind sharp. It turns your food into mental energy and repairs your brain tissue. Deficiencies in the B vitamins can cause mental functions. The way you make sure you get enough vitamin B in your diet is to eat foods containing rich grains, such as, breads, cereals, pasta, along with meats (3oz chicken breast, 3oz pork tenderloin and 3oz lean ground beef) Vitamin B6 is abundant in bake potatoes, bananas, turkey, and chickpeas.

Vitamin C

- **Vitamin C is good for the prevention of cancer.** Vitamin C has been shown to help prevent cancer causing compounds from forming in the digestive tract. It helps the small intestines absorbs iron. The body also uses vitamin C to produce collagen. Collagen helps to heal cuts and wounds.
- **Vitamin C is good for colds and flu.** Vitamin C strengthens white blood cells, which are essential for fighting off infections. Vitamin C has been shown to relieve cold symptoms by reducing the level of histamine, a naturally occurring chemical that makes your nose run.
- **Vitamin C is good for your immune system**. The most powerful protection for your immune system is to eat a well balanced diet which consists of fruits, vegetables, seeds and nuts, and seafood. These foods are high in nutrients that can keep your immune system healthy. The body uses vitamin C to make interferon, a protein that helps destroy viruses in the body. Vitamin C may also increase levels of a compound called glutathione, which has been shown to keep the immune system strong.

Vitamin D

- As bones get older it's essential to get extra calcium and vitamin D to prevent them from becoming brittle.

Vitamin E

- Vitamin E has gotten a lot of attention for its role for boosting immunity. The body uses vitamin E to produce a powerful immune protein called interleukin-2, which has been shown to tackle everything from bacteria and viruses to cancer cells.
- Vitamin E protects your fat tissues from free-radical invasion.
- Vitamin E is effective in the fight against heart disease. Vitamin E, which dissolves in fat, plays a powerful role in keeping your bad LDL cholesterol from oxidizing and contributing to atherosclerosis.
- Vitamin E works more efficiently when combined with vitamin C. After vitamin E becomes oxidized by free radicals, vitamin C comes along and regenerates it so that it's ready to work again. It's like vitamin C helps vitamin E get back on its feet again.

Antioxidants

Antioxidants are so important for your body. Antioxidants may help give the immune system a boost. You may ask why antioxidants are so important? The immune cells in your body are hit by a barrage of free radicals, harmful oxygen molecules that are created in great numbers every day. Since free radicals are missing an electron, they rush through your body, stealing electrons where ever they find them. And every time they grab an electron, another cell is damaged. The antioxidants in foods such as brightly colored fruits and vegetables literally come between free radicals and healthy immune cells, offering up their own electrons.

This neutralizes the free radicals by stopping them from doing further harm.

In one large study, researchers at the University of Helsinki in Finland reviewed 21 smaller studies that looked at how well vitamin C was able to beat colds. They found that people getting 1,000 milligrams of vitamin C a day were able to shorten the duration of their illnesses and reduce their symptoms by 23 percent.

Even though vitamin C is a powerful antioxidant it helps the immune system to destroy viruses in the body and to help keep the immune system strong. The best sources of antioxidants compounds are all fruits and vegetables. Foods such as cooked broccoli, butternut squash, strawberries, papaya, cantaloupe, oranges, baked sweet potato, sweet red pepper and watermelon. All vitamins are a good source of antioxidants for your body, especially vitamin C and vitamin E.

Oh my! We can't leave out coffee. Researchers found that no other food or beverage comes close to providing as many antioxidants in our diets as coffee. Of all the fruits and beverages studied, dates have more antioxidants per serving than coffee. Coffee in moderation is fine. One or two cups a day can be helpful. Did you know that coffee has been linked to decrease the risk of Parkinson's disease? The antioxidants in coffee may help protect against diabetes and colon cancer as well as regular and decaf coffee. It offers the same amount of antioxidants.

Detox fast if you've had too much coffee. You will know it by the twitch in your muscles or a flush on your face. To flush the caffeine out of your system, you should drink plenty of water.

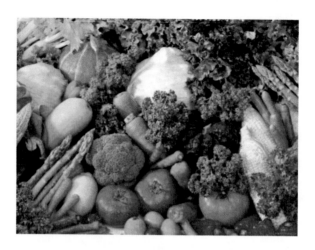

Chapter 3
Choosing your foods wisely will promote better health for your body, and can help you live a healthy lifestyle.

Diabetes

The fuel that keeps our bodies running is sugar, called glucose. Glucose pours into the bloodstream and is carried to individual cells throughout the body, soon after we eat. Before it enters in the cells, it requires a hormone called insulin. People with diabetes don't produce enough insulin, or the insulin they produce doesn't work efficiently.

Type 1 diabetes is the most serious form of diabetes. It occurs when the body makes little or no insulin. People with type 1 diabetes have to take insulin to replace their own insulin. Type 2 diabetes is more common. People with this condition may take oral medications, and don't require insulin injections, not during the early stages of this disease.

You need to fuel up with carbohydrates. Carbohydrates are the body's main source of energy. There are two types of carbohydrates. Simple carbohydrates, called sugars, include natural sugars found in milk, fruits, vegetables, and honey. Complex carbohydrates, called starches, include foods such as beans, potatoes, rice, and wheat pasta. The body turns simple and complex carbohydrates into glucose, which is converted into energy or stored up until the body needs it.

A high-fiber diet relieves constipation to heart disease. Fiber plays a role in controlling blood sugar. There are two types of fiber. Soluble and insoluble fiber plays a role in stabilizing blood sugar. Soluble fiber forms a gummy gel in the intestine, which helps prevent glucose from being absorbed into the blood too quickly.

Get help from vitamins. Two important vitamins for diabetes are vitamins C and E. If you have diabetes, fruits and vegetables rich in vitamins C and E are good for healthier eyes, blood vessels, and nerves. These vitamins are known as antioxidants. They help protect your body cells from free radicals. Oranges and grapefruits are excellent sources of vitamin C. But they are not the only ones. Tomatoes, cantaloupe, red peppers, and broccoli. Vitamin E, which is good for the heart is important for people with diabetes. Vitamin E help keeps blood platelets, which are elements in the blood that makes it clot, from becoming too sticky. To get the most vitamin E, use oils rich in polyunsaturated fats like, soy bean oil, corn oil, and sunflower oil. They will help boost your vitamin E level. Other good sources of vitamin E include sweet potatoes, blueberries, almonds, avocados, and kale.

Hypertension (high-blood pressure)

High blood pressure can make arteries in your brain
rupture or develop blockages leaving you disabled.
High blood pressure is bad on your kidneys and eyes. It
can put you on a dialysis machine and cause blindness.
Blood pressure can go up or down during the course of
the day. Your heart pumps blood throughout your body
sending blood through your arteries. Each time your
heart beats, it sends out a new wave of blood that
makes your blood pressure to go up. This is called your
systolic blood pressure. Your heart briefly relaxes
between beats and the pressure subsides. This is called
your diastolic blood pressure. You kidneys, brain,
heart, and eyes, and other organs depend on a reliable
blood flow.

Blood with high pressure goes through the arteries with
a damaging force. The heart has to struggle harder to
push out the blood, and could grow enlarged and unable
to bear the extra strain. Your arteries may grow stiff
and narrow. This sends less blood to your organs and a
blood clot can block the flow, causing a heart attack.

Being overweight or obese, having a diet that provides
too much salt or too little potassium, excessive alcohol
use, chronic stress, causes high-blood pressure. This
life style can be preventable. Give your heart a break
by losing weight. Losing weight can reduce your blood
pressure or prevent you from developing hypertension.
The best weight loss diet is to eat low-fat foods, and eat
lots of fruits and vegetables, with exercise.

Cholesterol

The body uses cholesterol which is produced in the liver, to make cell membranes, sex hormones, bile acids, and vitamin D. In large amounts, found in animal foods such as meats, eggs, milk and butter are dangerous for your body. Having high cholesterol levels is one of the primary risk factors for heart attack, and strokes. Elevated cholesterol puts you at higher risks for heart disease. Eating foods that are low in saturated fats and cholesterol is an efficient way to reduce the amount of cholesterol in your blood. Making small reductions in cholesterol can add up to big health benefits.

What are the good and bad types of cholesterol?

Low- density lipoprotein (LDL) is bad cholesterol. The more LDL you have in your blood stream, the higher your risk for heart disease. High-density lipoprotein (HDL) is good cholesterol. This type lowers your risk for heart disease.

Triglycerides are another type of fat in your blood. People with diabetes and those who are at risk of diabetes tend to have high triglycerides. When you make changes in your lifestyle to improve your cholesterol levels, you want to lower LDL, raise HDL, and lower triglycerides.

You may ask what are the best ways to improve your cholesterol?

- **Eat more fish**. Oily fish such as salmon, tuna, sardines, and mackerel, are best. Fish that are caught in the wild are better for you than fish that are raised on farms. You should eat one or two 6oz servings each week.
- **Eat more nuts.** Have a hand full of nuts, such as, almonds, pecans, walnuts, hazelnuts, or brazile nuts once a day instead of unhealthy snacks.
- **Eat less saturated fats.** There are two kinds of saturated fat. One is in animal products and some plant foods (coconut and palm kernel oil). The other kind is a man -made saturated fat called trans fat. Trans fats are used in margin and many snack foods.
- **Eat more unsaturated fats.** Most fats in vegetables, tree nuts, grains are unsaturated. There are two kinds of unsaturated fats (monounsaturated and polyunsaturated). These are better for you than saturated fats.
- **Eat more high-fiber foods.** Good sources include beans, whole oats, vegetables, whole grains, peas, and flax seed.
- **Eat more soy protein.** Get more protein from plant sources, such as soy, instead of meats. Soy protein shakes are an easy way to add soy to your diet.
- **Fish oil.** If you don't eat fish regularly, you can take fish oil supplements with at least 1,000 mg of fatty acids EPA and DHA.

Alzheimer's disease

Alzheimer's disease is a form of dementia, which

causes a decline in mental abilities. When people have this condition, portions of the brain shrivel up and shrink, twisted tangles of protein develop within the brain cells, and other deposits of protein develop between the brain cells.

Since there is no cure for Alzheimer's, researchers are focusing their attention on nutrition. Research has uncovered evidence that free radicals, which are harmful oxygen molecules that damage tissues throughout the body, including the brain, may play a role in Alzheimer's disease. Even though the body produces a protective substance called antioxidants that help control free-radicals, the body needs more antioxidants by simply eating more fruits and vegetables that contain antioxidant substances.

Researchers are also investigating B vitamins as a way of treating Alzheimer's disease. The body uses B vitamins to help maintain the protective covering on nerves and to manufacture chemicals that nerves use to communicate. When levels of B vitamins decline, mental performance may suffer, says Dr. Penland. A diet rich in fruits and vegetables, fish, whole grain, unsaturated fats such as olive oil, may help protect you from Alzheimer's disease.

Good sources of thiamin, a B vitamin include sunflower seeds, pork, and enriched grain products. For vitamin B12, seafood such as sardines, tuna, steamed clams, and meats such as lamb, chicken livers, and turkey are all good sources. For folate good sources include enriched cereals. For B6 vitamin eat some bananas, potatoes, Chicken, and chickpeas.

Headaches

Headaches are caused by certain foods we eat. The nitrites that are used to preserve cured meats such as bologna, hot dogs, hog head cheese, and meats packaged in a can may cause blood vessels in the head and body to dilate with pain. And monosodiume glutamate (MSG) a flavor enhancer and a preservative that's used in a variety of foods including Chinese food, lunch meats, canned soups, and frozen dinners, can cause headaches.

There are two types of headache pain. Muscle contraction or tension headache, and migraine headache is called vascular headache. This type of headache is caused by contraction of blood vessels in the face, head, and neck. Both tension and vascular headaches can be caused by stress, hormone levels, or either the changes in the weather. But the substances that are found in foods are to be blamed.

Strokes

Strokes occur when blood, oxygen and the nutrients it contains, stop reaching parts of the brain. Usually to a blood clot blocking a tiny artery in your brain or, less often, when an artery ruptures and blood is lost. The most frightening thing about a stroke is how suddenly it can strike. High blood pressure, high cholesterol, diabetes and a dangerous pre-diabetic condition called metabolic syndrome all raise your risk. They are all factors that can be reduced by choosing healthy foods.

Your diet plays a critical role in preventing a stroke, says Thomas A. Pearson, MD, PhD.

High blood pressure doubles your risk for a stroke. Why? Because high speed blood flow, arteries in the brain thicken and can ultimely squeeze shut. Small arteries may rupture under pressure. High blood pressure elevates the risk for developing clot-producing plaque in artery walls. Include low-fat dairy products and plenty of potassium-rich foods in your diet. Potassium fights high blood pressure by making blood less likely to clot, which reduces the risk of a stroke. Foods that are good sources of potassium are fat free and 1% milk, low-fat yogurt, vegetable juice cocktail, lentils, baby lima beans, baked potatoes, dried peaches, prune juice, and kidney beans.

Reverse metabolic syndrome by choosing to eat smart. Metabolic syndrome is a combination of pre-diabetic conditions including insulin resistance, which occurs when your cells stop responding to insulin's command to absorb blood sugar. Plus slightly high blood sugar, high blood pressure, and triglycerides. Nearly everyone with this condition is overweight. Having metabolic syndrome doubles the risk of having a stroke.

What fights it? Eating fruits and vegetables, high fiber, low sugar foods, good fats such as nuts, lean protein, oily cold water fish (or fish oil capsules), and flax seed. Eating fruits, vegetables, and grain products low on the glycemic index also keeps your blood sugar and insulin level lower. This cuts cravings and helps you lose weight. Foods to avoid are doughnuts, sugary soft drinks, and white bread, which send sugar level rising fast. Foods to embrace are most whole grains, beans, fruits and vegetables, which digest more slowly and so release sugar into the blood stream at a regular rate.

Lose weight. Not only what you eat but how much you eat can play a role in controlling a stroke. Being overweight can raise a woman's stroke risk by 75%. Obesity raises it by 100%. Being overweight is perhaps the leading cause of high blood pressure, which increases the risk of having a stroke. People with high blood pressure are five times likely to have a stroke than those who have normal blood pressure. Also, being overweight makes you more likely to develop diabetes, which also increase the risk of having a stroke.

Choose lots of produce, too. There are several reasons that fruits and vegetables are so beneficial for preventing a stroke. First, they are high in fiber, which has been shown to lower cholesterol. Foods that are high in antioxidant include onions, carrots, blueberries, cherries, garlic, Brussels sprouts, red grapes, oranges and broccoli. Along with fruits and vegetables, tea (green& black) is an excellent source of flavonoids.

Heart Attacks (disease)

Healing power of a Mediterranean diet can help reduce the risk of heart disease. The Mediterranean diet emphasizes seasonally fresh and locally grown fruits and vegetables over processed foods that don't contain antioxidants. Fresh fruits serve as a dessert while sweeter deserts are consumed no more than a few times a week. People who eat the most fruits and vegetables have fewer problems with heart disease. This is due to the antioxidant vitamins and other healing compounds in these foods.

The Mediterranean diet is high in fiber. High fiber foods help keep your weight down by filling you up without a lot of fat and calories. High fiber foods help block the absorption of certain fats and cholesterol. This means that some of these harmful substances are flushed away before making it into the bloodstream. In addition, fruits, vegetables, and beans which are another Mediterranean staple, are among the best sources of folate, a B vitamin that may work hard in the fight against heart disease, says Dr. Gardner.

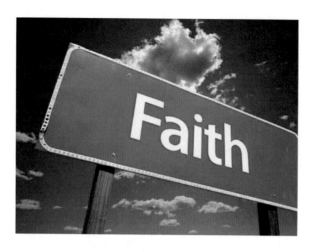

Chapter 4

Faith

I would like to thank God for allowing me to write this book with confidence, courage, and Faith. For without faith it is impossible to please God. Faith is putting your trust in God in all things. Faith is having a personal relationship with God knowing and believing that nothing is impossible or to hard for God. Know that we can do all things through Christ who strengthens us. If you have the faith the size of a mustard seed you can move mountains in the name of Jesus. That mountain can be depression, oppression, addiction, low-self esteem, financial problems, relationship problems, marriage problems, family problems, lying, cheating, beating your way through life, stealing, bad eating habits, stress, obesity, heart disease, diabetes, high-blood pressure, bad cholesterol, and all evil works and acts of the devil.

The problems you face everyday, such as, stress,

depression, oppression, financial problems, bill
collectors calling every hour of the day, marriage
problems, relationship problems, obesity, diabetes, bad
cholesterol level, high-blood pressure, and family
problems are enough to take a toll on your body. Next
thing you know, your chest is feeling tight, you are
having a fierce headache, shortness of breath, feeling
dizzy and nausea. Your children are acting out (getting
on your last nerve), the wife is always fussing and
clowning about every little thing, (it seems like you
can't do anything right). Her main concern is getting
her husband to live a healthy lifestyle by eating healthy,
and getting her husband to go to the doctor to get a
complete physical so he can live longer.

The Epistle of James says, "Faith without works cannot
be called faith". "Faith without works is dead"(2:26),
and dead faith is worse than no faith at all. Verbal faith
is not enough; mental faith is insufficient. Faith must be
there, but it must be more. It must inspire action.
Through his epistle to Jewish believers, James
integrates true faith and everyday practical experience
by stressing that true faith must manifest itself in works
of faith.

Faith endures trials. Trials come and go, but a strong
faith will face them head-on and develop endurance.
Faith understands temptations. It will not allow us to
consent to our lust and slide into sin. Faith obeys the
word. It will not merely hear and not do. Faith
produces doers. Faith harbors no prejudice. For James,
faith and favoritism cannot coexist. Faith displays itself
in works. Faith is more than mere words; it is more
than knowledge; it is demonstrated by obedience; and it

overtly responds to the promises of God. Faith controls the tongue. This small but immensely powerful part of the body must be held check. Faith can do it. Faith acts wisely. It gives us the ability to choose wisdom that is heavenly and to shun wisdom that is earthly. Faith produces separation from the world and submission to God. It provides us with the ability to resist the Devil and humbly draw near to God. Finally, Faith waits patiently for the coming of the Lord. Through trouble and trial it stifles complaining.

Now is the time to put your best foot forward with faith, in fighting to live a healthy lifestyle. You can put your best foot forward with faith by:

- **Praying**

- **Worshiping**

- **Daily bible reading**

- **Seeking God in all things**

- **Changing your eating habits**

- **Drinking plenty of water**

- **Walking**

- **Getting plenty of sleep**

By faith we understand in Hebrews 11: 1-3: Now faith is the substance of things hoped for, the evidence of